YOUR KNOWLEDGE HAS VALUE

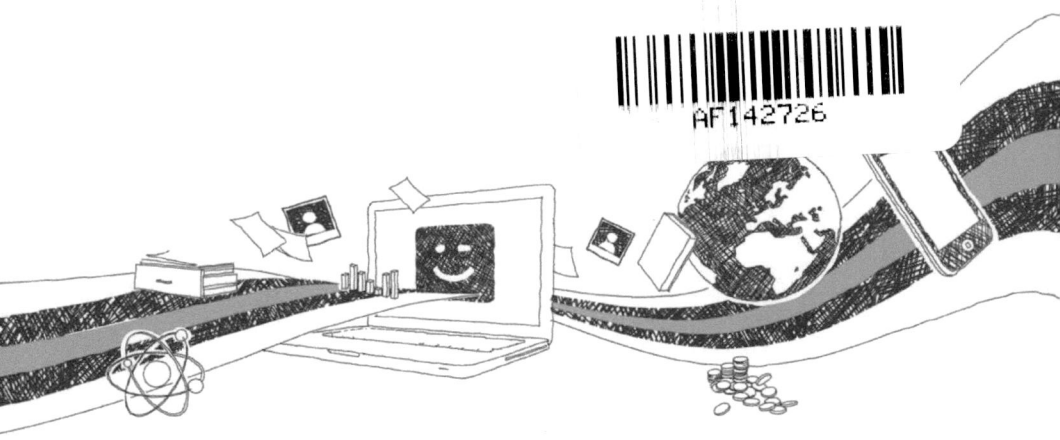

- We will publish your bachelor's and master's thesis, essays and papers

- Your own eBook and book - sold worldwide in all relevant shops

- Earn money with each sale

Upload your text at www.GRIN.com and publish for free

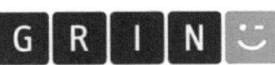

Bibliographic information published by the German National Library:

The German National Library lists this publication in the National Bibliography; detailed bibliographic data are available on the Internet at http://dnb.dnb.de .

Imprint:

Copyright © 2017 GRIN Verlag
Print and binding: Books on Demand GmbH, Norderstedt Germany
ISBN: 9783346173034

This book at GRIN:

https://www.grin.com/document/517311

Paul Mutale, Patrick Mbewe

Socioeconomic Determinants of Malaria among Children in Zambia

GRIN Verlag

GRIN - Your knowledge has value

Since its foundation in 1998, GRIN has specialized in publishing academic texts by students, college teachers and other academics as e-book and printed book. The website www.grin.com is an ideal platform for presenting term papers, final papers, scientific essays, dissertations and specialist books.

Visit us on the internet:

http://www.grin.com/

http://www.facebook.com/grincom

http://www.twitter.com/grin_com

THE UNIVERSITY OF ZAMBIA

SCHOOL OF HUMANITIES AND SOCIAL SCIENCES

DEPARTMENT OF ECONOMICS

TOPIC: SOCIOECONOMIC DETERMINANTS OF MALARIA INCIDENCES AMONG CHILDREN UNDER FIVE IN ZAMBIA

PATRICK MBEWE
PAUL SAMPA MUTALE

A Research Report submitted in partial fulfillment of the requirements for the Award of the Bachelors of Arts Degree in Economics.

ABSTRACT

There are wide gaps in empirical information on socioeconomic determinants of malaria among children under five. The main objective of this study was to investigate the socioeconomic factors such as mother's education level, wealth of household, age of child, employment status and gender of child among other variables to establish how they influence malaria in children under five years of age.

Initially a proportional cross-sectional analysis was conducted using the 2013/14 Zambia demographic health survey report (ZDHS) data. The results of proportion of children who had malaria by their socioeconomic characteristics were highest among children aged 12-23 months with malaria of 27.1 percent prevalence levels while across child gender about 20.4 percent males and 21.6 percent females had malaria . In relation to mothers education highest proportions were observed among mothers with no education representing 24 percent with lowest 15percent for those with more than secondary school level of education. In terms of wealth the highest proportion was observed from second and lowest wealth quartile with 23.6 and 22.7 percent respectively while the lowest 17.6 percent was observed from those in the highest or richest level of wealth.

Then a probit regression analysis was done among selected socioeconomic factors and marginal effects where computed and presented in table 5, the probit regression show that a total of 9722 observations were analyzed and that if the average age of a child in months goes up by one unit, the probability of a child having malaria reduces by 0.078%. In terms of education mothers who have had no education increases the probability of a child having malaria by 3.22% holding other variable constant. This is a clear indication of the influences of socio economic factors on prevalence of malaria in children under five.

ACKNOWLEDGEMENT

We would like to extend our deepest appreciation to our supervisor Dr. Jolly Kamwanga for his tireless direction and guidance that forged this study. We further acknowledge the Director of National Malaria Control (NMC) Dr. H. Busiku for his guidance and most importantly our Lecturer Dr. C.M Chiliba and Mr. B. Chizonde for their general guidance on how to conduct the study. We also recognize the invaluable contributions to this study by the entire team from the Department of Economics of the University of Zambia and our fellow students. Special gratitude to all respondents for finding time to interact with this study in their classes and offices hence enabling its completion, May God bless them abundantly.

Above all, we absolutely indebted to the Almighty God for the gift of life and health we undeservedly enjoyed throughout the period of our studies.

ABBREVIATIONS

MOH:	Ministry of health
NMCC:	National malaria control Centre
MOJ:	Ministry of Justice
WHO:	World health organization
IRS:	Indoor residual spraying
ITN:	Insecticide treated nets
ZDHS:	Zambia demographic health survey
MIS:	Malaria indicator survey
HMIS:	Health management and information system
RDT:	Rapid diagnostic test
IMCI:	Integrated management of childhood illness
ITGFHW:	Integrated technical guidelines for frontline health workers

TABLE OF CONTENTS

1.0.0 INTRODUCTION

1.1.0 Background

Malaria is an entrenched global health challenge particularly in the sub-Saharan African countries. An estimated 219 million cases of malaria and 660,000 malaria deaths occurred worldwide in 2010, (WHO: World malaria report, 2012). Approximately 80% of malaria episodes and 90% of the deaths were reported from the African continent according to the 2012 world malaria report. Endemic malaria results in tremendous economic losses annually and is a central element of the vicious cycle of poverty in many developing countries. International funding for malaria control rose to a peak of USD 1.84 billion in 2012,World malaria report (2012) . The world malaria report of 2011 shows an estimated 655,000 malaria deaths in the world, majority of which were under-five children from Africa . Thus, it remains a leading cause of death in children under five years (Sutcliffe CG, 2012). The World Health Organization and United Nations Children's Education Fund (UNICEF, 2008) also indicate in the African Malaria Report that over 3,000 children die from malaria in Africa daily with a child dying every 30 seconds.

Malaria prevention and control in Zambia commenced in 1952. Since then great progress have been achieved, however, malaria still kills more children under the age of five than any other disease. It affects more than 4 million Zambians annually (UNICEF, 2008), causing 30% of outpatient visits resulting into about 8000 deaths each year. Under five children and pregnant women are most vulnerable with 35 to 50 percent child mortality and 20 percent maternal mortality, (Asenso-Okyere, 2003). Overall, the 2012 malaria indicator survey MIS shows that malaria parasite prevalence was 14.9% with more parasitaemia among children in rural areas (20.2%) compared to urban areas (13.7%). On average, parasitaemia prevalence peaked among children aged four years and was highest in Luapula province (32.1%) and in the lowest wealth quintile (27.4%), (MIS, 2012).

Malaria parasite rates typically increase with increasing age in the first five years of life (MIS, 2012). A number of studies have been conducted on malaria among under-five children and had attributed the disease to nonuse of insecticide treated nets (ITNs) by care givers among other studies have also conducted studies on malaria related beliefs and behaviors, treatment, prevention, and control in Southern and western provinces. However, little research has been done on socioeconomic determinants of malaria in Zambia. As such, this study sought to examine the socioeconomic factors that determine malaria among under-five children in Zambia using the latest cross sectional data from the 2013/14 Zambia demographic survey report.

1.2.0 Problem Statement

Malaria is endemic both in urban and rural areas. It is documented as the most common cause of out-patient attendance and hospital admission in all age groups in Zambia (Kalubula M, 2016). Malaria is associated with the socio-economic status (SES) of countries. Given the extent of malaria in southern Africa, a full understanding of the factors associated with malaria incidence is important. This study will examine to what extent social and economic factors influence malaria episodes in households in children under five using the 2013/14 Zambia demographic survey data. Most studies have focused on the effectiveness of scientific methods of interventions such as indoor residual spraying, insecticide treated nets and Intermittent preservative treatment while other researchers have focused on the determinants of ITN use or factors influencing demand for IRS very few knowledge is linked to the social economic factors that determine malaria in children under five. This study intends to add education of the mother, wealth, age, sex, area and to establish the probability of children having malaria.

1.3.0 Justification

There is need to fully understand the determinants of malaria in order to reduce the burden that malaria puts on the health care system as well as the economic system. Being endemic in sub-Saharan Africa, there is need for adequate information about malaria for effective health policies to be put in place. Policies that the poor countries and communities can afford are vital as they will be easy to implement, compared to policies that require the intervention of donors.

Studies carried out previously show that the environment (temperature, humidity and rainfall), behaviour and demographic factor also an important driver of malaria (Bennett, 2013). Determining the spatial distribution of malaria is also important in ensuring that areas with high incidence are prioritized in the distribution of resources as well as in malaria prevention programs.

This study will give insight as to what are some of the socioeconomic factors that increase the chances of under five children to have malaria as such change the perception of policy makers from the business as usual syndrome in the fight against malaria.

1.4.0 GENERAL OBJECTIVES

The general objective of the study was to describe and analyze social and economic determinants of malaria incidence among children under five years in households in the Zambian population of 2014.

1.5.0 Specific Objective

❖ To investigate the determinants of malaria episodes in children under five years in Zambia.

❖ To investigate the extent to which social and economic factors influence malaria episodes among children under five

❖ To investigate and compare proportional distribution of malaria episodes among socioeconomic factors.

1.6.0 Research Question

❖ What are the socioeconomic factors associated with malaria?

❖ How is malaria distributed across socio economic status in children?

❖ What relationship exists between factors and malaria in children?

❖ To what extent do the determinants affect the occurrence of malaria in children under five?

1.7.0 Hypotheses Statements

❖ Socioeconomic factors have no influence on malaria episodes among children under five

❖ Wealth of household has no influence on malaria in children under five

❖ Mothers education has no influence on malaria in children under five

1.7.0 Significance of study

❖ The findings can be used as empirical evidence regarding the influence of socioeconomic factors on malaria occurrence among under five children

❖ The findings can be used as a basis for policy formulation in the fight against malaria

❖ The findings will add to the existing literature and general body of knowledge

1.8.0 Scope of Study

This study focuses on an inquiry on the socioeconomic determinants of malaria in children under five years of age in Zambia. There are other factors that influence prevalence of malaria in children; these include demographic factors such as age, sex, ethnicity and environmental factors like temperature, humidity, climate etc. Our study seeks to use secondary data from the 2013/14 Zambia demographic health survey (ZDHS) to establish the social and economic factors that influence malaria in children such as mother's education , child age, child gender , region of residence and economic factors such as wealth of household. We will cover the sample of under five children surveyed in the ZDHS which was done at national level.

1.9.0 Limitation

This study relies on secondary data obtained from the ZDHS report. We could not conduct primary data collection because time and resource constraints. In order to access data a formal request was made on 30th July, 2017 to the Program Demographic Health Survey (PDHS) world data where access was granted on 2nd August, 2017 specific to the our research topic. Therefore, we had no control as to what extent the data we need was to be made available for instance the only variable which closely relates with malaria in children was a question of fever in the last two weeks , the data set did not have precise information on the malaria test results in children under five years, consequently, fever in the last two weeks was used as proxy to explain malaria in children since by definition all fever above 38.5 degree Celsius in children must be treated as malaria this was the case definition in Zambia and many sub-Saharan African countries before the introduction and availability of rapid diagnostic tests or in absence of malaria confirmation procedures.

Finally money was a major constraint as movement to meet with our supervisors required transport. The last minute new regulations by national malaria control center requiring a medical approval form delayed our data collection process.

2.0.0 LITERATURE REVIEW

2.1.0 Malaria in Zambia

Zambia is one of the unique countries that have experienced down and upward swing in the prevalence of malaria in the past 60 decades. Prior to 1970, malaria in urban areas in Zambia, especially towns along the line of rail (Copper, Lusaka to Livingstone), was kept to a minimum due to effective implementation of prevention and control programme (MoH, 2007). Vector control, especially IRS, was at its highest in the local, municipal and mine controlled towns and this contributed to reduction in malaria incidence. Konkola copper mines effectively carried out IRS, which resulted in reduction of incidence rate from 68/1000 to 20/1000 for Chingola and 158/1000 for Chililabombwe respectively, (Chanda E, 2011).

In addition, according to the Health Information Management System, HMIS (2010-2015) data, malaria incidence in Zambia increased from 230/1000 cases in 2010 to 335/1000 cases in 2015. These variations in incidence rates show a general increase in malaria cases at national level. However,

4

notable increase and decreases has been observed in some provinces the largest relative decline in parasite prevalence by microscopy was observed in Luapula Province (51% - 32%), 2010 to 2012 HMIS data. North-Western Province had the largest relative increase in parasite prevalence (6% - 17%), while Northern Province remained relatively unchanged (24%). HMIS (2010-2012).

Malaria can be defined as a protozoan infection of the genus Plasmodium, transmitted through the bite of an infected female mosquito belonging to the genus Anopheles (MoH, 2000)Plasmodium falciparum is a protozoan parasite, one of the species Plasmodium that causes malaria in humans, transmitted by the female Anopheles mosquito. Under 5 child means a child whose aged 0–5 years.

2.2.0 Malaria transmission and illness

Malaria is caused by four species of parasites of the genus Plasmodium that affect humans (P. falciparum, P. vivax, P. ovale, and P. malariae). Malaria is mainly found in tropical Introduction areas(Mendis and Carter, 1995). Malaria due to P. falciparum is the most dangerous form and it is mainly found in Africa; P. vivax is less dangerous but more widespread, and the other two species are found much less frequently (WHO: World malaria report, 2012). P. falciparum is responsible for almost all the malaria mortality cases in Sub-Saharan Africa and it is often stated that the continent bears over 90 percent of the global P. falciparum burden (Snow and Omumbo, 2006). Malaria infection is caused by mosquito bites and manifests itself in different ways. Severe malaria can result in severe anaemia, respiratory distress in relation to metabolic acidosis, or cerebral malaria. In adults, multi-organ involvement is also frequent. Immunity may develop in malaria endemic areas, resulting in mild infections to occur, particularly in adults. No clinical syndrome is entirely specific for malaria, (Ayeni, 2011).

2.3.0 Factors associated with malaria illness

Malaria transmission is controlled by environmental factors which affect the intensity of distribution, seasonality and transmission (Alegana, 2006). Malaria thrives in conditions that promote the growth of the vector of malaria which is the mosquito. Studies have shown that a dirty environment can result in increased malaria transmission (Sutcliffe CG, 2012). Other factors are temperature, humidity, rainfall, forest clearance, agriculture and non-availability of insecticide treated mosquito nets (Eisele TP, 2012), rainfall leaves pools of stagnant water that are good breeding for mosquitoes, clearing of forests results in light being able to penetrate into the forest and therefore providing ideal breeding for mosquitoes and in Zambia, firewood is the main source of fuel (Chanda E, 2011). This leads to the destruction of forests and thereby promoting mosquito breeding. Agricultural methods that involve irrigation as well as the building of dams also promote the breeding of mosquitoes therefore these results in increased malaria transmission (Abeku, 2003). All these factors promote malaria illness as these result in increased chances of a person being bitten by mosquitoes.

Another study suggested that, socio-economic status (SES), immunization, knowledge, human behaviour and general under nutrition also play a role in increasing malaria illness and mortality. Nutrition is linked to economic status if one is economically sound then they are able to provide adequately for themselves and therefore resulting in a well-nourished body. A well-nourished body is immune competent to fight off malaria infection by mounting an adequate response to infection as compared to an immune vulnerable undernourished body (Eisele TP, 2012). Malaria severely affects nutrition by limiting food intake through lack of appetite and vomiting; Nutritional status also affects responses to anti-malarial medication (Bates, 2004) resulting in drug resistance. Approximately 67% of anaemia cases in children in malaria-endemic countries are thought to be the result of malaria (Bates , 2004). Health status is also linked to economic status and malaria is also affected by the economic status of an individual as well as country (Asenso-Okyere, 2003). A poor economic status results in inadequate health care facilities in Zambia and therefore increasing vulnerability of the population to malaria. A review of literature on SES and malaria showed that malaria and low SES were interlinked.

Age and gender are the other important factors that are also associated with malaria illness with the majority of malaria illness and deaths occurring in children under the age of five. Studies carried out in Gabon and Tanzania showed that children over the age of five were most at risk in the transmission of malaria (D. Houeto, 2007; Eisele TP, 2012). In the Tanzania study, males were more at risk of malaria illness compared to females, (Kim D, 2012). A study carried out in rural Nigeria did not show any difference between the sexes but showed that prevalence of malaria was highest in 11 to 20 years age group (Ayeni, 2011). Another study carried out in Kenya showed that parasitaemia decreased with age with children in the 1-4 year age group having the highest prevalence at 83% and decreasing to 60% in the 10-14 year age group (Brooker, 2008). In Zambia it has been shown that malaria increase with age and that children under five carry the heaviest burden of malaria, the parasite rates typically increase with increasing age in the first five years of life this is because their immune system is not yet fully developed, (Chizema-Kawesha E, 2010).

Studies also suggest that location also plays an important role in malaria transmission. In one study carried out in Ethiopia, clustering or hot spots of malaria were revealed (Abeku, 2003). Another study carried out in Ghana showed that distance from a water body plays an important role in malaria prevalence (Asenso-Okyere, 2003).

2.4.0 Conceptual Framework

The conceptual framework table 1 , shows the relationship of socioeconomic factors on malaria.

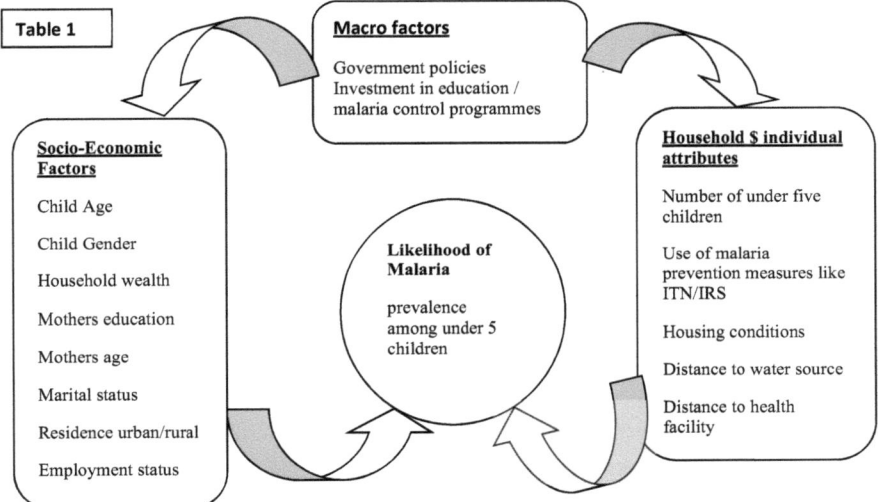

3.0.0 METHODOLOGY

This paper used secondary data drawn from the 2013/14 Zambia Demographic and Health Survey (ZDHS) children's data file. The ZDHS is a national sample survey designed to provide up to date information on background characteristics of the respondents, fertility levels, sexual activity, fertility preferences, awareness and use of family planning methods, breastfeeding practices, nutritional status of mothers and young children, early childhood mortality and

maternal mortality, maternal and child health, awareness and behaviors regarding HIV/AIDS and other sexually transmitted infections (STIs), and prevalence and incidence of HIV/AIDS and other STIs. The target groups were men age 15-59 years and women age 15-49 years in randomly selected households across Zambia, (Phiri, 2013). Information about children age 0-5 years was also collected, including data on weight and height. The survey collected blood samples for HIV testing in order to determine national and provincial prevalence and incidence rates. The Question for malaria incidence and prevalence data was collected on children who reported to have had fever in the past 2 weeks before the survey diagnostics test where not conducted.

The ZDHS was carried out by the Central Statistics office (CSO), the ministry of health (MoH), the University of Zambia Teaching Hospital (UTH) Virology Laboratory, the Tropical Diseases Research Centre (TDRC), and the Department of Population Studies at the University of Zambia (UNZA), (CSO, MOH, ICF international, 2015).

3.1.0 Sample design

The sample for the 2013-14 ZDHS was designed to provide estimates at the national and provincial levels, as well as for rural and urban areas within the provinces. This is the first time the ZDHS has been designed to provide estimates at such disaggregated levels for many of the survey indicators. The updated list of enumeration areas (EAs) for the 2010 Population and Housing Census provided the sampling frame for the survey. The frame comprises 25,631 EAs and 2,815,897 households. A representative sample of 18,052 households was drawn for the 2013-14 ZDHS. The survey used a two-stage stratified cluster sample design, with EAs (or clusters) selected during the first stage and households selected during the second stage. In the first stage, 722 EAs (305 in urban areas and 417 in rural areas) were selected with probability proportional to size. Zambia is now administratively divided into 10 provinces (Central, Copperbelt, Eastern, Luapula, Lusaka, Muchinga, Northern, North Western, Southern, and Western). Stratification was achieved by separating each province into urban and rural areas. Therefore, the 10 provinces were stratified into 20 sampling strata. In the second stage, a complete list of households served as the sampling frame in the selection of households for enumeration. An average of 25 households was selected in each EA. It was during the second stage of selection that a representative sample of 18,052 households was selected. Data collection took place over an eight-month period, from August 2013 to April 2014. (Central statistics office, 2015).

Out of a total of 18,052 households selected from 722 clusters 16,258 were occupied at the time of the fieldwork and 15,920 of the occupied households were successfully interviewed, yielding a household response rate of 98 percent. In the interviewed households, a total of 17,064 women age 15-49 were identified as eligible for individual interviews, and 96 percent of these women were successfully interviewed. A total of 16,209 men age 15-59 were identified as eligible for interviews, and 91 percent were successfully interviewed. Generally, Individual response rates were slightly lower in urban areas than in rural areas.

The survey obtained information on women's exposure to malaria during their most recent pregnancy in the five years preceding the survey and the treatment for malaria. They were also asked if any of their children born in the five years preceding the survey had malaria, or fever in the last two weeks prior to survey and whether these children were treated for malaria, and about the type of treatment they received.

In this study fever in the last two weeks was used as a surrogate for malaria firstly because the data set from ZDHS had no information on the test results for malaria in children under five. Secondly malaria is the leading cause of fever in Sub-Saharan Africa, where 30 to 60% of fevers especially in infants and young children are attributed to malaria (Mabunda S, 2009). In highly endemic areas, fever alone is used as a proxy for symptomatic malaria it was applied in a study in Mozambique where a report of fever in last 30 days was associated with confirmed Rapid diagnostic testing RDT results. In Zambia Fever is a major manifestation of malaria and other acute infections in children. Malaria contributes to high levels of morbidity and mortality. While fever can occur year-round, malaria is more prevalent following the end of the rainy season. In the past, malaria treatment guidelines as well as the ITG guidelines were based on the assumption that fever on its own was an indication of malaria, in line with the then-prevailing epidemiological pattern of malaria in the country (CSO, MOH, ICF international, 2015). As such Medical personnel used this method to diagnose patients especially if they have no means to conduct confirmatory tests such cases are reported as clinical malaria and treatment is given (Chirwa, 2002, p. 69) . However, it must be acknowledged that while report of fever approximates symptomatic malaria, it underestimates malaria prevalence in children especially in the rainy season. The statistical package STATA (version 12) was used to process the data.

3.2 Variable definition; table 2

Type of variable	Variable name	Variable definition
Dependant variable	Malaria	Fever/malaria in child under five in last two weeks 0=no had no malaria 1=yes had malaria
Independent variable	Region	**Categorized** Provinces: Lusaka, northen, southern, eastern, western, luapula central, muchinga, copperbelt,N/western
	Residence	1=urban 0=rural
	Mothers education	Highest level of education attained categorical Variable
	Married	Marital status 1=yes 0=no
	Wealth	Is wealth index of household 1=poorest 2=poorer 3=middle 4=richer
	Itn_use	Slept under mosquito net last night 1=yes 0=no
	Child gender	Sex of a child 1=male 2=female

3.3.0 Model estimation Technique

In this study we used probit model to conduct our analysis and the model specifications are;

Probit (p=1 if malaria present or otherwise =0)

$P(Y=1|X_{1i},...,X_{ki}) = \Phi(B0 + B1 \text{ child\_ageMth} + B2 \text{ region} + B3\text{edu\_year} + B4\text{no\_childunder5} + B5\text{wealth} + B6 \text{ married1} + B7\text{religion} + B8 \text{ child\_gdr} + B9 \text{ irs} + B10 \text{ itn\_use5} + B11 \text{ residenc})$

$Y = \Phi(X\beta + u)$ the value of X is taken to be the standard normal variables, Φ where if then $\Phi \sim N(0, \sigma^2)$.

Where $F(\Phi)$ is the cumulative distribution function(CDF) of the normal distribution and

(u) is the stochastic term where we assume var(u^2)=1, $\sigma^2=1$

$P(Y = 1 \mid X)$ means the probability that an event occurs given the value(s) of the X, or explanatory, variable(s) and therefore the CDF will be

$$F(\Phi) = \int_{-\infty}^{\Phi} \frac{1}{\sqrt{2\pi \, \sigma^2}} \, e^{-\frac{1}{2\sigma^2}(x-u)^2 dx}$$

3.4.0 Justification for choice of probit model

Probit model is type of regression where the dependant variable can take only the two values, for example child has malaria=1 or child has no malaria=0. The purpose of the model is to estimate the probability that an observation with particular characteristics will fall into one category. Therefore the probit regression model was used because of asymmetric distribution of data in terms of malaria cases and the fact that the outcome variable has a binary response denoting whether or not a child had malaria. In addition Probit model is chosen in this study because of the large sample size of observation over 9000 observations and we assume that the error term is normally distributed hence will use Z-score for testing hypothesis.

4.0.0 FINDINGS

4.1.0 Introduction

In this section will show the findings of the research by presenting a table of proportional analysis done to show the distributions of malaria cases within the various selected variables. Hence, results were presented in frequencies and proportions. Then a table of diagnostic test done prior to adoption of the model is presented. Finally a probit regression model was applied to study the factors that determine malaria cases among children under five. This was done by adding factors in stages in order to identify consistent and robust predictors of malaria, and then robust probit regression was conducted due to heteroscedasticity problem. In order to interpret the effects of the predictors' marginal effects were computed and presented. Some of the independent variables especially categorical variables marital status, wealth and employment were modified to suit the study while some were used as they were found in the original dataset. Thereafter a discussion, conclusion based on findings and recommendations were made.

4.2.0 Data presentation

4.2.1 Proportional presentation of malaria distribution across selected factors

Table 3 below shows the results of proportion of children who had malaria by their socioeconomic characteristics. The highest prevalence of malaria of 27.1 percent was among children aged 12-23 months malaria was lowest with 12 percent among children less than 6 months and 15percent for those aged between 48-49 months. About 20.4 percent males had malaria while 21.6 percent were females. In relation to residence 18.6 percent were malaria in children living in urban and while 22.3 percent rural. Malaria prevalence was highest with in northern province 26 percent north western 23.8 percent and lowest in Lusaka with 15.3 percent. Highest proportions of malaria were also observed among mothers with no education representing 24 percent with lowest 15percent among mothers who have had more than secondary school level of education.

In terms of wealth the highest proportion was observed from second and lowest wealth quartile with 23.6 and 22.7 percent respectively while the lowest 17.6 percent was observed from those in the highest or richest level of wealth.

Table 3: proportion of malaria among under 5 children

	Percentage With malaria	number of children
Age in months		
<6	12.6	1,204
6-11	25.3	1,274
12-23	27.1	2,575
24-35	23.9	2,507
36-47	19.9	2,447
48-59	15.1	2,627
Sex		
Male	20.4	6,393
Female	21.6	6,240
Residence		
Urban	18.6	4,318
Rural	22.3	8,316
Province		
Central	18.6	1,241
Copperbelt	19.5	1,634
Eastern	22.6	1,603
Luapula	23.1	1,112
Lusaka	15.3	1,855
Muchinga	22.8	771
Northern	26.0	1,203
North Western	23.3	641
Southern	21.2	1,754
Western	23.8	821
Mother's education		
No education	24.2	1,387
Primary	21.1	7,098
Secondary	20.3	3,696
More than secondary	15.7	453
Wealth quintile		
Lowest	22.7	3,032
Second	23.6	2,905
Middle	20.9	2,604
Fourth	18.5	2,208
Highest	17.6	1,884
Total	**21.0**	**12,634**

Source: computed from ZDHS 2013-14

Generally malaria has been observed to be highest among children aged 12-23months, those found in rural areas and by region it is more common in northern, north western, western provinces. Mothers with least or no education have many children with malaria which is similar with the wealth quartile factor where the poorest or lowest wealth quartile highest malaria among under five children.

Then prior to the probit analysis we present a summary of diagnostic test done leading to choice of the variables of interest in our model as shown in the table 2 below.

4.3.0 Summary of Diagnostic Test

Table 4: Diagnostic test done on the probit regression model

No	Test command	Purpose of test	Acceptance rule	Results	Remark
1	Estat class	Model fit	Correctly classified if >50%	77.79% > 50%	Passed test, Model is correctly classified therefore correctly fits the data
2	Linktest	Model specification	_hat must be significant; P-value < 0.05	P-value hat 0.006	Passed test, model is correctly specified
			_hatsq must be insignificant; P-value >0.05	P-value hatsq 0.110	
3	Vif, uncentered	multicollinearity	Vif must be < 10	Mean vif 2.88 ; Max vif 5.56 ; Min vif 1.14	Passed test, no multicollinearity problem
4	Hetprob	heteroscedasticity	Prob > chi2, P_value > 0.05 means there is no heteroscedasticity	wealth2 Prob > chi2 = 0.0054 (no_childu5) Prob > chi2 = 0.0002 (medu1)Prob > chi2 = 0.0121 (medu4) Prob > chi2 = 0.0315 (child_ageMth)Prob > chi2 = 0.0003	Model failed the test, Therefore we have a problem of heteroscedasticity. In order to control this problem we will run robust probit model

From the test done findings show that child age, wealth and mothers education are associated with heteroscedasticity problem. To solve this problem we opted to run the White's Heteroscedasticity-Consistent Variances and Standard Errors regression also known as the robust standard errors. In addition due to model specification and multicollinearity problem we dropped some variables earlier suggested in our model estimation technique and included new ones in order to have well specified model which has no multicollinearity problem. Dropped variables include region, residence, religion, indoor residual spraying in household (irs) and insecticide treated net use among children (itn_use).

Included variables in categorical employed and not employed, time taken to water source, (ttws), wealth and mothers education in category form.

4.4.0 Probit Regression Model With Robust Standard Errors

The probit regression model with robust standard errors was done based on the notion that that it as has been shown that this estimate can be performed so that asymptotically valid large-sample statistical inferences can be made about the true parameter values and it is viable option where weighted least squares method could not be done (Domadar N. Gujurati, 2009). This regression shows the adjusted standard errors but the slope coefficient does not indicate the effect of variables on the likelihood of a child having malaria. The probit regression model required 4 iterations to obtain the psuedo log likelihood ratio of -5100.69 however, the estimated coefficients do not quantify the influence of the independent variables (x) on the probability that malaria the dependant variable takes on the value one, the estimated coefficients are parameters of the latent model. As such in this study we run the (mfx compute) command after running the probit model with robust standard errors and presented the marginal effect regression table in order to interpret the effect of socioeconomic factors on prevalence of malaria among children.

4.5.0 Marginal effects of probit analysis

4.5.1 The extent of socioeconomic factors influence on malaria

Table 5 below shows the slope coefficients as the influence that each independent variable has on the probability of children under five having malaria. The marginal slope coefficients represent the extent to which socioeconomic factors influence the probability of malaria prevalence among children. Therefore the effect of a unit change of the independent variable on the probability $P(Y = 1|X = x)$, given that all other regressors are constant. It is vital to note that with binary independent variables, marginal effects measure discrete change, such as how predicted probabilities change as the binary independent variable changes from 0 to 1. Marginal effects for continuous variables measure the instantaneous rate of change in the independent variable and how it affects probability of children having malaria.

Therefore from table 5 below, if the average age of a child in months changes by an infinitesimal amount, the probability of a child having malaria reduces by 0.078% while holding all other variables constant (ceteris Paribas). In terms of education mothers who have had no education (medu1) increases the probability of a child having malaria by 3.22%, ceteris Paribas .While mothers who have had higher education (medu4) that is above secondary school level reduces that chances of a child having malaria by 5.91%, ceteris Paribas . In addition if the average number of children five and under, (child_ageMth), in a family changes by an infinitesimal amount the probability of a child having malaria reduces by 2.1%, ceteris Paribas. The wealth category indicate that if a household is poor,(wealth2) the probability of a child having malaria increases by 2.96%, ceteris Paribas.

Table 5 ; marginal effects of probit regression model

```
. mfx compute

Marginal effects after probit
      y  = Pr(malaria) (predict)
         =  .21986213
```

variable	dy/dx	Std. Err.	z	P>|z|	[95% C.I.]	X
child_~h	-.0007844	.00024	-3.32	0.001	-.001247 -.000321	29.2383
medu4*	-.0590758	.02277	-2.59	0.009	-.10371 -.014442	.036309
medu1*	.0321838	.01394	2.31	0.021	.004859 .059508	.111808
no_chi~5	-.0207541	.00508	-4.09	0.000	-.030706 -.010802	1.96348
male*	-.0042945	.00842	-0.51	0.610	-.020798 .012209	.501543
wealth2*	.0296128	.01034	2.86	0.004	.009346 .049879	.237605
wealth5*	-.0287084	.0141	-2.04	0.042	-.056342 -.001075	.126311
ttws	-.0000823	.00017	-0.47	0.636	-.000423 .000258	18.1741
married*	-.0135531	.01146	-1.18	0.237	-.03601 .008904	.833265
employ~3*	.0033978	.01789	0.19	0.849	-.031661 .038457	.562744
notemp~1*	-.0480231	.01789	-2.68	0.007	-.083094 -.012952	.378317

```
(*) dy/dx is for discrete change of dummy variable from 0 to 1

.
```

Where, as if the household falls in the richest category, (wealth5), the probability of a child having malaria reduces by 2.87%, ceteris Paribas. If the respondent was not employed (notemployed1), the probability of a child having malaria reduces by 4.8% while those employed had statistically no influence on the probability of children having malaria.

4.6.0 Hypothesis testing

We conducted hypothesis testing based on the P-value of variables. If P-value < 0.05 then the variable is significant otherwise it is insignificant

❖ **Ho:** Socioeconomic factors have no influence on occurrence of malaria in children under 5
  Ha: Socioeconomic factors have influence on occurrence of malaria in children under 5
  Wealth, age of child, mothers education, employment were found to be statistically significant at 5% level thus we reject Ho and conclude that socioeconomic factors do influence occurrence of malaria among under five

❖ **Ho:** Wealth of household has no influence on malaria in children under five
  Ha: Wealth of household has influence on malaria in children under five

Wealth was found to be significant poor(wealth2) P-value 0.004 < 0.05, richest(wealth5) P-value 0.042 < 0.05, therefore we reject Ho and conclude that wealth has influence on malaria in children under five

❖ **Ho:** Mothers education has no influence on malaria in children under five
  Ha: Mothers education has influence on malaria in children under five
  Mothers with no education (medu1) P-value 0.021 < 0.05; significant
  Mother with higher education (medu4) P-value 0.009 < 0.05 significant
  Therefore we reject Ho and conclude that mother's education has influence on malaria in children under five.

5.0.0 DISCUSSION

5.1.0 Socio economic factors influencing malaria among children under five

This study proposed that socioeconomic factors determine the prevalence of malaria in children under five. From our findings the following factors were statistically significant at 5% confidence level which means that we are 95% confident that they influence the likelihood of malaria among children, these include age of child, number of under five children in a household, mothers education, wealth of household and employment status of head of household.

5.1.1 Statistically significant factors

Age of a child

Age of a child has influence on the likelihood of having malaria as the findings indicated a reduction in the chances as the child grows. It must also be noted from the proportional distribution of malaria that prevalence reduces with increase in age there could be more to this phenomenon than just age which may hint on a child having stronger immunity, behaviour change because as the child grows, they tend to be more aware of the environment as well as easily communicate with their parents.

Number of under 5 children in household

According to our findings an increase in number of children under age five has negative relationship or reduces the probability of a child having malaria by a very small margin of 0.078%. This small reduction implies that more than likely large population of children under five may increase chances of malaria among them. This is related to other factors such wealth because typically poor families are associated large family size, low education and high unemployment levels. Therefore there is need to perceive malaria as complex disease which requires integrated strategies to combat it.

Mother's education

Mother's education statistically indicated that mothers with no education increase the chances of children having malaria unlike those who attained secondary school or higher. These findings enlighten us on the importance of education and provoke thoughts of advocating for improvement in that area. In Zambia, It has been attributed that mothers mostly spend time with their children compared to their male spouse, this implies that even the level of care for the children could be attributed to how well the mother relate to environment around her. This includes, understanding health education information given by the ministry of health such as using protective measures against mosquito bites and seek early treatment for any ailments. Others may argue that health education is delivered in simplest form and local language but that is just a mode of communication. Mothers education is vital as it enhances the mothers ability to cognitively act on information made available to them, by keeping in check of all necessary measures required to ensure their children are healthy.

Wealth

Wealth of household indicated that it was significant in influencing the probability of a child having malaria. Poor household, both from the proportional table and marginal effect analysis statistically indicate that they increase the probability of children having malaria. This means poor families are more likely to have children with malaria than rich families. These observations echo the assumption that malaria is a disease of the poor. Therefore the richer a household is the less likely malaria would occur among under five children.

Employment status of head of household

When we relate education level and wealth we realize that both low education level and low wealth increase likelihood of malaria in children. Education cost money and thus requires a certain level of wealth and wealth creation requires individuals to engage in some form of occupation or being employed. These factors seemingly unrelated but are related to some extent. From our marginal effect analysis employed head of house has statistically no influence on malaria in children under five. However, those unemployed seem to reduce chances of children having malaria. This variable does not make practical sense however these were the results of the finding.

5.1.2 Statistically insignificant factors

Child gender (male), marital status (married), time taken to water source (ttws) and those employed where insignificant variables in our analysis. This means they have statistically no effect on the probability of a child having malaria.

5.2.0 Conclusion

It is clear from our findings that statistically wealth, mother's education, number of under five children in a household, age of child and employment status influence the probability of children having malaria. Therefore we reject the null hypothesis that socioeconomic factor do not affect occurrence of malaria in children under five. However in relations to marital status (married), male gender of the child; and time taken to water source, have no influence on the chances of malaria among children

This empirical analysis provides a basis for further investigations in the relationships between malaria and socio economic factors. Policy makers should look into an inclusive approach to the fight against malaria because of the complex nature of the problem among children. The use of conventional methods has proved effective in some areas but even that success is married with factors like wealth and mothers education. Lusaka is highly industrialized province it is not surprising that such places have low proportions of malaria unlike north western , western, Luapula and northern provinces where there is very low industrial activities. Therefore it is not necessarily about region in this case or climatic conditions because Zambia enjoys fairly similar climatic conditions everywhere but rather it borders on the socio and economic conditions prevailing in a household.

5.3.0 Recommendations

The following are suggested recommendations made for policy makers to consider in their bid to fight against malaria among children;

- ❖ Policy makers targeting elimination of malaria should include malaria prevention education in school curriculums
- ❖ The government apart from focusing on treatment indoor residue spraying and itn distribution should increase expenditure in education and champion girl child education. Because the same girls become mothers in the future.
- ❖ Government should focus on wealth creation activities and developmental projects among its citizens such as empowering youths on merit with soft loans to run business
- ❖ Government and parents should discourage early marriages as these deter women from attaining higher levels of education
- ❖ More research to be done on social economic factors influencing malaria and other diseases or attenuating conditions
- ❖ Governments should plan some special polices to improve female education like introducing special stipends for female students and also making education free at least up to secondary school level even though this may mean heavy taxes to finance expenditure
- ❖ It is also necessary for governments to the economic environment favorable for local investors by encouraging domestic consumption to enable wealth creation.

6.0.0 REFRENCE

- Abeku, T. A., Van Oortmarssen, G. J., Borsboom, G., De Vlas, S. J. & Habbema, J. D. F. (2003), Spatial and temporal variations of malaria epidemic risk in Ethiopia: factors involved and implications. Acta Tropica 87, 331-340.

- Ademowo, O., Falusi, A. & Mewoyeka, O. (1995). Prevalence of asymptomatic parasitaemia in an urban and rural community in south western Nigeria. The Central African journal of medicine, 41, 18-21.

- Akazili, J., Aikins, M. & Binka, F. N. (2008) Malaria treatment in Northern Ghana: What is the treatment cost per case to households? African Journal of Health Sciences, 14, 70-79.

- Alegana, V. A., Atkinson, P. M., Wright, J. A., Kamwi, R., Uusiku, P., Katokele, S., Snow, R. W. & Noor, A. M. (2013). Estimation of malaria incidence in northern Namibia in 2009 using Bayesian conditional-autoregressive spatial–temporal models. Spatial and spatio-temporal epidemiology, 7, 25-36.

- Alegana, V. A., Wright, J. A., Nahzat, S. M., Butt, W., Sediqi, A. W., Habib, N., Snow, R. W., Atkinson, P. M. & Noor, A. M. (2006). Modelling the Incidence of Plasmodium vivax and Plasmodium falciparum Malaria in Afghanistan 2006–2009. PloS one, 9, e102304.

- Ayeni, A. (2011). Malaria morbidity in Akure, southwest Nigeria: A temporal observation in a climate change scenario. Trends in Applied Sciences Research, 6, 488-494.

- Bates, I., Fenton, C., Gruber, J., Lalloo, D., Lara, A. M., Squire, S. B., Theobald, S., Thomson, R. & Tolhurst, R. (2004). Vulnerability to malaria, tuberculosis, and HIV/AIDS infection and disease. Part 1: determinants operating at individual and household level. The Lancet Infectious Diseases, 4, 267-277.

- Ben chirwa (2002) integrated technical guideline for frontline health workers; editon 2 pg 62

- Bennett, A., Kazembe, L., Mathanga, D. P., Kinyoki, D., Ali, D., Snow, R. W. & Noor, A. M. (2013), Mapping malaria transmission intensity in Malawi, 2000-2010. Am J Trop Med Hyg, 89, 840-9.

- Bloland, P. B., Boriga, D. A., Ruebush, T. K., Mccormick, J. B., Roberts, J. M., Oloo, A. J., Hawley, W., Lal, A., Nahlen, B. & Campbell, C. C. (1999). Longitudinal cohort study of the epidemiology of malaria infections in an area of intense malaria transmission II epidemiology of malaria infection and disease among children. American Journal of Tropical Medicine and Hygiene, 60, 641-8.

- Breman, J. G., Alilio, M. S. & Mills, A. (2004) Conquering the intolerable burden of malaria: what's new, what's needed: a summary. The American journal of tropical medicine and hygiene, 71, 1-15.
- Brooker, S., Clarke, S., Snow, R. W. & Bundy, D. A. (2008). Malaria in African schoolchildren: options for control. Trans R Soc Trop Med Hyg, 102, 304-5.
- Chanda E, Hemingway J, Kleinschmidt I, Reman A, Ramdeen V, Phiri FN, Coetzer S, Mthembu D, Shinondo CJ, Chizema-Kawesha E, Kamuliwo M, Mukonka V, Baboo KS, Coleman M (2011): Insecticide resistance and the future of malaria control in Zambia. PLoS One, :e24336.
- Chanda E, Masaninga F, Coleman M, Sikaala C, Katebe C, MacDonald M, Baboo KS, Govere J, Manga L (2008): Integrated vector management: the Zambian experience. Malar J, 7:164.
- Chizema-Kawesha E, Miller JM, Steketee RW, Mukonka VM, Mukuka C,Mohamed AD, Miti SK, Campbell CC: (2010) Scaling up malaria control in Zambia:progress and impact 2005–2008. Am J Trop Med Hyg, 83:480–488.
- CSO, MOH, ICF international, (2015) Zambia Demographic Health survey 2013-14, rockville, maryland: CSO
- D. Houeto, W. D'Hoore, E. Ouendo, D. Charlier, and A. Deccache,(2007) "Malaria control among children under five in sub-Saharan Africa: the role of empowerment and parents' participation besides the clinical strategies," Rural and Remote Health Journal, vol. 7, no. 4, article 840,
- Domadar N. Gujurati, D. C. P., (2009), Basic Econometrics. 5th edition ed. New york: McGraw-Hill/Irwin
- Eisele TP, Larsen DA, Anglewicz PA, Keating J, Yukich J, Bennett A, et al. (2012) Malaria prevention in pregnancy, birthweight, and neonatal mortality: a meta-analysis of 32 national cross-sectional datasets in Africa. Lancet Infect Dis.;12:942–9.
- Kalubula M, L. Q. S. G. L. X., (2016). A District Level Linear Regression Analysis of Malaria Morbidity and. Epidemeology, 6(2)
- Kalubula M, L. Q. S. G. L. X., (2016.) A District Level Linear Regression Analysis of Malaria Morbidity and. Epidemeology, 6(2.
- Killeen GF, Smith TA, Ferguson HM, Mshinda H, Abdulla S, Lengeler C, Kachur SP (2007): Preventing childhood malaria in Africa by protecting adults from mosquitoes with insecticide-treated nets. PLoS Med , 4:e229
- Kim D, Fedak K, Kramer R(2012). Reduction of malaria prevalence by indoor residual spraying: a meta-regression analysis. Am J Trop Med Hyg. ;87:117–24.

- Mabunda S, C. S. A. J. T. A. A. P., (2009). A country wide malaria survey in mozambique. malaria Attributable proption of feverand establishment of malaria case definition in children in children accross diffrent epidemiological settings., p. 8:74

- Mabunda S, Casimiro S, Apontte JJ, Tiango A, Alonso P (2009), A country wide malaria survey in Mozambique ;malaria Attributable proption of fever and establishment of malaria case definition in children in children accross different epidemiological settings. page8:74

- Ministry of Health (2001): Roll Back Malaria Strategic Plan (2001–2005) Ministry of Health, Lusaka;

- MIS, (2012) malaria indicator survey report for 2012,; national ,national malaria control center,Lusaka

- MoH, (2000). National malaria situation analysis report., lusaka: Ministry of Health

- NMCC (2011): Zambia national malaria control program performance review. Lusaka, Zambia: National Malaria Control Centre, Ministry of Health;.

- Phiri, E., (2013) Effect Of Indoor Residual Spraying On Incidence Of, Lusaka: S.N.

- Sutcliffe CG, Kobayashi T, Hamapumbu H, Shields T, Mharakurwa S, Thuma PE, Louis TA, Glass G, Moss WJ (2012): Reduced risk of malaria parasitemia following household screening and treatment: a cross-sectiony6y6665...al and longitudinal cohort study. PLoS One 2012, 7:e31396.

- UNICEF, (2007) Zambia Fact Sheet: Malaria,; UNICEFUnited Nations Children's Education Fund

- United Nations Children's Education Fund,(2007),UNICEF Zambia Fact Sheet: Malaria

- Utzinger J, Tozan Y, Doumani F, Singer BH (2002),: The economic payoffs of integrated malaria control in the Zambian copperbelt between 1930 and 1950. Trop Med Int Health 7:657–677.Watson M, J. M., 1953. The battle for health in central Africa. 1 ed. london: African highway.

- Watson M: African highway(1953).: The battle for health in central Africa. London:John Murray;

- WHO: World malaria report (2012). Geneva: World Health Organization, Available from: http://www.who.int/malaria/publications/

- WHO: World malaria report, (2012) World Health Organization, world malalria report , Geneva:

YOUR KNOWLEDGE HAS VALUE

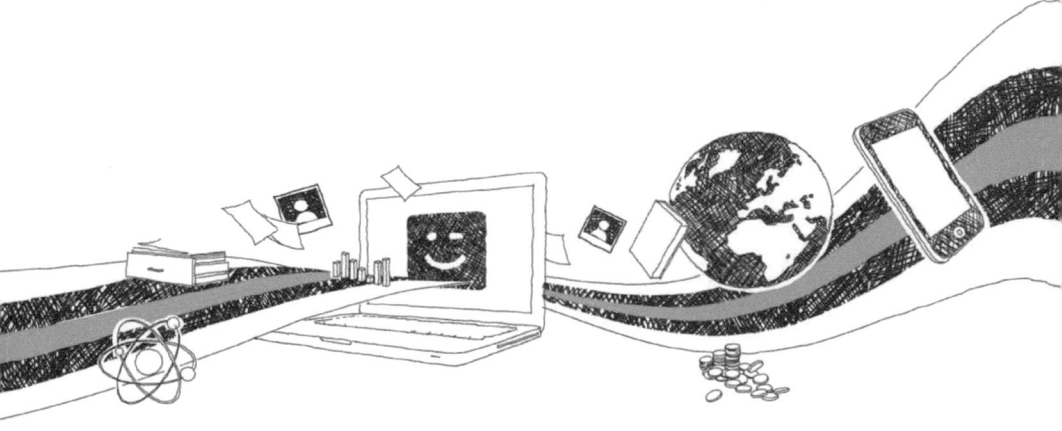

- We will publish your bachelor's and master's thesis, essays and papers

- Your own eBook and book - sold worldwide in all relevant shops

- Earn money with each sale

Upload your text at www.GRIN.com
and publish for free

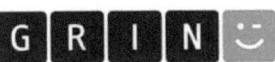